ELENA R. MONTIRES

30 Bodyweight Exercises

Build Strength at Home Without Equipment

Introduction

Welcome to the world of bodyweight training! Here we will discover the power of using only your own body as a fitness tool. In this world of a sedentary lifestyle and huge amounts of stress, maintaining a healthy body is a struggle for many people. Having access to quick fixes, gadgets, and trending workout fads, we can be distracted from the true essence of exercise. The beauty of bodyweight training is that we only need one fitness tool, OURSELVES!

These exercises can be completed anywhere, including your home, backyard, the park, and at any time since they require no equipment but your own body! This makes these exercises perfect for anyone who is on a budget or just has a busy lifestyle with no time to make it to the gym.

In this book, you will find two sections of exercises broken up into different categories: Upper Body Exercises, Lower Body Exercises, and Core Exercises. You can use these exercises to create your own fitness regimen, depending on what areas of the body you would like to workout.

These exercises are just a starting point for your fitness journey! Remember, there are always different ways to modify each exercise, take it at your own pace, and stay hydrated. Below you will find the benefits of Bodyweight Exercises, How to Use This Book, Warm Up/Cooldown Guidelines, and Safety Precautions. Please make sure to read and understand all sections before creating your own workout regimen and beginning your fitness journey.

Benefits of Bodyweight Exercises

Convenience

The biggest benefit of bodyweight training is that no matter where you are, you always have your body with you! This means you can complete a bodyweight workout wherever you are, at whatever time you have available.

Price

Since there is no additional equipment needed, this type of training is perfect for those looking to get fit on a budget.

Location

These exercises can be completed anywhere! If you prefer to be at home by yourself, you can! Or if you want to be outside, take it to the backyard or your local park. Also, if you feel intimidated in the gym atmosphere of machines and bodybuilders, this is a great way to avoid that intimidation. Complete these exercises in the comfort of your own home with nothing to be intimidated by.

Modifications Available

It may not seem obvious at first but, all bodyweight exercises can be modified to your own fitness level. For each exercise we will provide modification options. Also, you can adjust the length of time or number of sets and/or reps you will complete during the regimen.

It Is Good For You

Many studies have shown that the more exercise you do, the lower the risk of diseases, obesity, joint pain, and more. Exercising can lift your mood, improve your sleeping habits, reduce stress, and much more!

How To Use This Book To Create Your Workout

Creating your own workout can be done in many different ways, but for the purposes of this book, we will focus on two methods: The Timed Method and The Sets and Reps Method. Please make sure to warm up before your workout and cool down after your workout to prevent injury.

The Timed Method

The Timed Method focuses on doing each exercise for a certain amount of time followed by a period of rest. This is called a round. Rounds can be made up of any number of exercises, though we suggest picking 5 different exercises per round, then completing 3 rounds. As you progress in your fitness journey you can adjust the number of exercises per round and the number of total rounds to challenge yourself.

Example Timed Method Exercise Focused on Lower Body: Do 30 seconds of five exercises with 15 seconds of rest between each exercise. Rest for 1 minute between each round. Complete 3 rounds, with a warm up before and a cool down after:

30 Seconds of Calf Raises, 15 Seconds Rest

30 Seconds of Squats, 15 Seconds Rest

30 Seconds of Side Leg Raises, 15 Seconds Rest

30 Seconds of Bridges, 15 Seconds of Rest

30 Seconds of Plank Jacks, 15 Seconds Rest

Rest for 1 minute before starting at the beginning and completing 3 more rounds.

The Sets and Reps Method

The Sets and Reps Method focuses on completing a certain number of sets and reps, rather than time. Rep is short for the word repetition. One rep is a single execution of an exercise. For example, one push up is one rep. A set can be anywhere between 8 to 12 reps. Please remember that if the exercise uses one leg at a time, one rep is the completion of both legs. For example, one rep of lunges is one lunge using your right leg and one lunge using your left leg.

Example Sets and Reps Exercise Focused on Lower Body Breakdown: Do each exercise for the amounts of reps and sets below with a small amount or rest between each set, with a warm up before and cool down after:

12 reps/ 3 sets Calf Raises (One rep is one Calf Raise)

12 reps/ 3 sets Squats (One rep is one Squat)

12 reps/ 3 sets Side Leg Raises(One rep is a Side Leg Raise with the right leg and one Side Leg Raise with the left leg)

12 reps/ 3 sets Bridges (One rep is Bridge)

12 reps/ 3 sets Plank Jacks (One rep is one Plank Jack)

Warm up/Cooldown Guidelines

Warm Up Guidelines

Warming up your body will help prevent injury by preparing your body for the exercise regimen ahead. An effective warm up will increase your body temperature, increase blood flow to your muscles, and may help reduce soreness. A warm up should last between 10 to 15 minutes. Focus on warming up the muscle groups you plan on activating during your workout as well as large muscle groups. Here are some examples of warm ups:

- To warm up for a lower body focused workout, do the exercises you will be doing in the workout in a slower fashion while focusing on engaging the muscles that will be used in your regimen (Slow Squats, Slow Lunges, Slow Calf raises, Etc)
- To warm up for an upper body focused workout, do the exercises you will be doing in the workout in a slower fashion while focusing on engaging the muscles that will be used in your regimen (Slow Arm Circles,Slow Push Ups, Slow Inchworms, Etc.)

Cooldown Guidelines

Cooling down your body will help prevent injury and can help prevent soreness. Your Cooldown should last anywhere between 5-10 minutes and should reduce your heart rate back down to a regular pace. Include stretching here to improve range of motion and flexibility. An effective way to cool down is to continue your workout, but in a slower and less intense fashion, then finish off with some stretching. Make sure to target the areas that were worked during your exercise.

Safety Precautions

When beginning a new exercise regimen, we tend to push ourselves too far and put ourselves at risk. Please make sure to listen to your body and modify your exercises when needed. Below are some tips to exercise safely:

- Stay Hydrated: Make sure to drink enough water to keep your body hydrated while exercising.
- ALWAYS Warm up and Cooldown: Doing your warm up and cooldown can help prevent injury.
- Dress Appropriately: Wear the appropriate clothing for the location and temperature you will be performing your exercises.
- Replace Your Shoes As They Wear Out: It is recommended to replace your shoes every 6 to 8 months, however, this can vary depending on the shoe material, type of workouts done, and location where the workouts are completed.
- Listen to Your Body: Listening to your body can help prevent injury. You will recognize your own limitations by listening to your body.

Please make sure to consult your physician before starting any exercise regimen for your safety.

Upper Body Exercises

Push ups

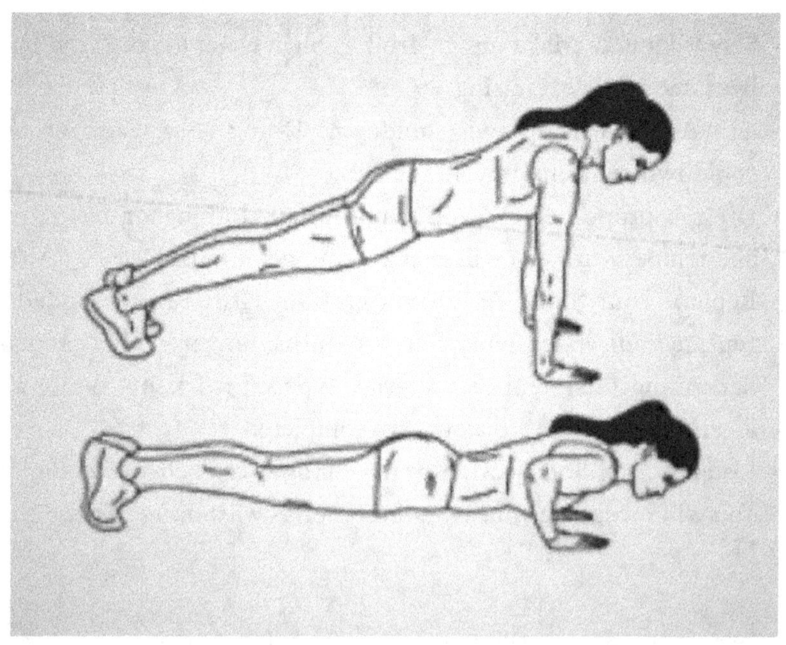

Push Ups

How to:

- Start at a prone position. Hands are in place under the shoulders with the elbows extended. Make sure to keep the legs straight with toes touching the ground. Lower the body by bending the elbows until the arms are parallel to the ground. Lastly, reverse the movement and push the body off the ground until back in the starting position. Make sure to keep the core tight for stabilization.

Modifications:

- Knee Push Ups: Place the knees on the ground instead of the toes
- Wall Push Ups: Place the hands on a wall instead of the ground

Muscles Being Worked:

- Chest
- Back
- Shoulders
- Arms
- Core

Upper Body Exercises

Shadow Boxing

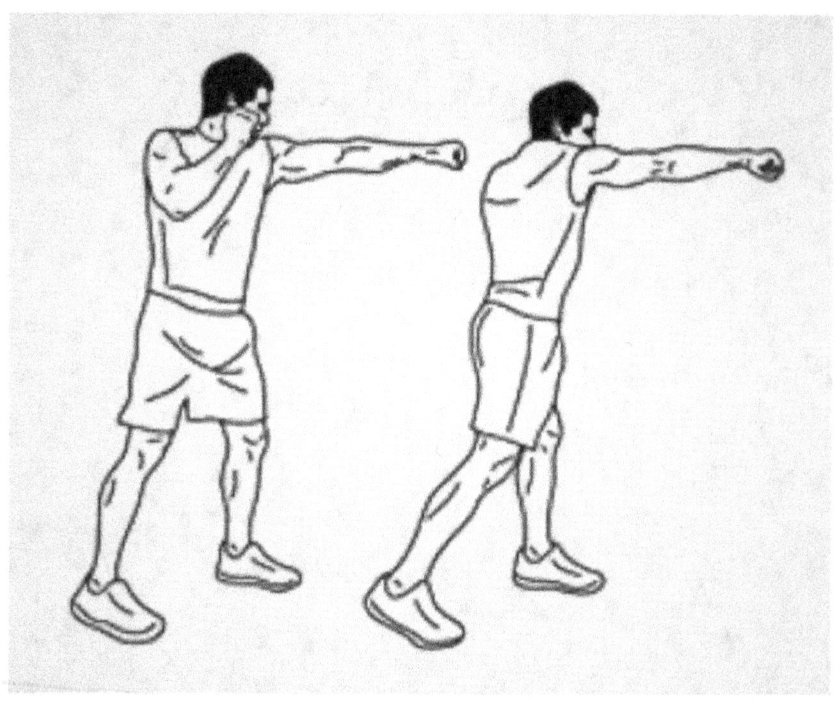

Shadow Boxing

How to:

- Get in a standing boxing stance and pretend there is an opponent in front of you. Then proceed to do any of the following moves, or make up your own combos. Make sure to keep the stance strong, core tight, and focus on every move:
- Jab, Cross
- Hook Right, Hook Left
- Elbow Strike Right, Elbow Strike Left

Modifications:

- Slower Combo Shadow Boxing
- Faster Combo Shadow Boxing

Muscles Being Worked:

- Chest
- Shoulders
- Arms
- Core
- Back

Upper Body Exercises

Arm Circles

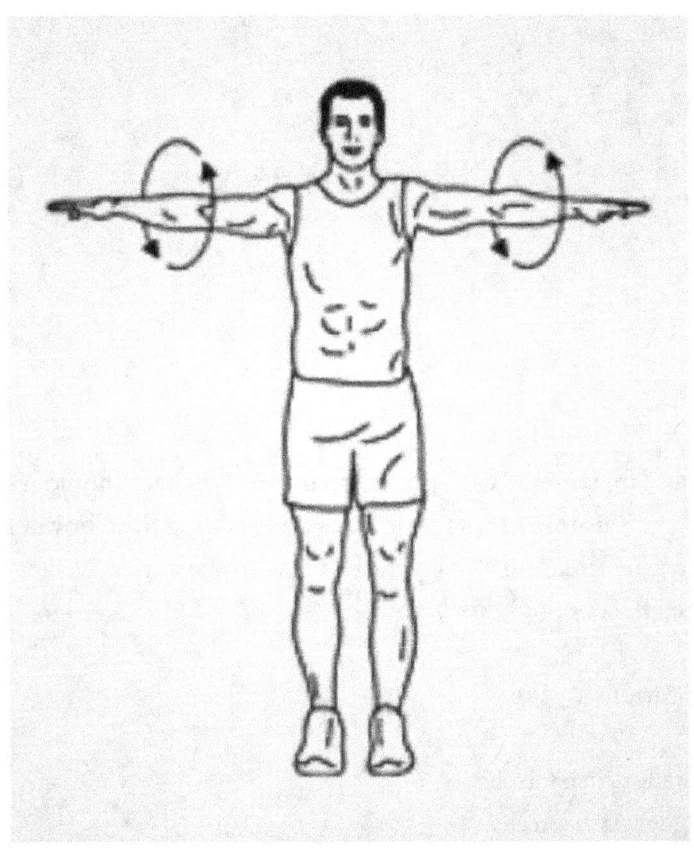

Arm Circles

How to:

- Stand up straight with good posture and the feet shoulder-width apart. Raise the arms to the sides not bending the elbows. Rotate the arms creating a circle in the air with the hands. Make sure to keep the core tight for stability.

Modifications:

- Smaller Arm Circles
- Bigger Arm Circles
- Slower Arm Circles
- Faster Arm Circles

Muscles Being Worked:

- Shoulders
- Arms
- Chest
- Back
- Core

Upper Body Exercises

Back Extension Pull Downs

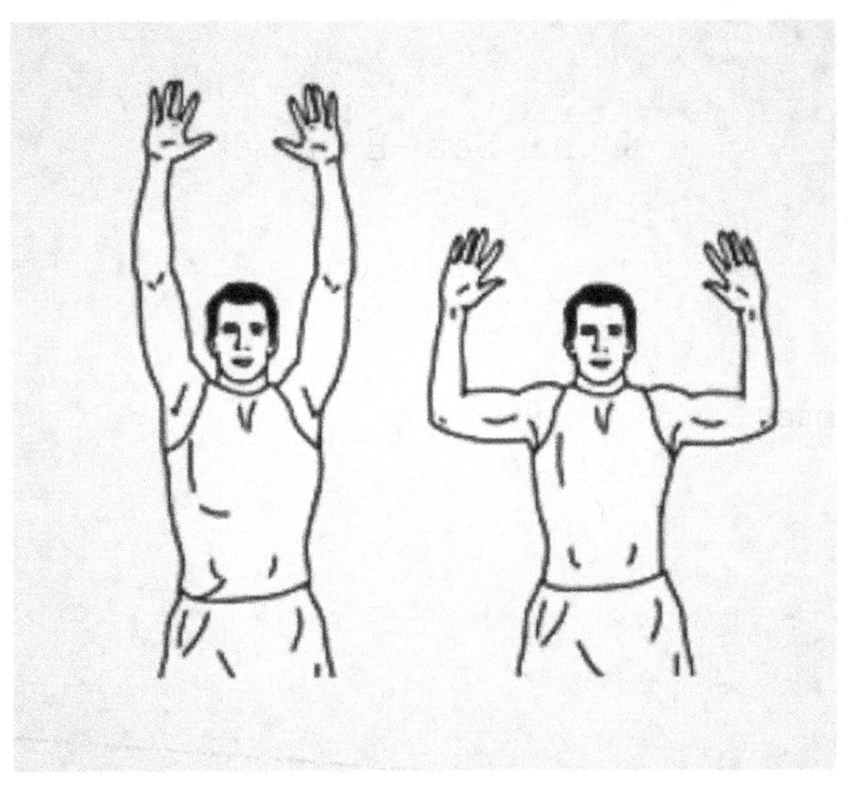

Back Extension Pull Downs

How to:

- Stand up straight with a good posture and the feet shoulder-width apart. Raise your arms above the head making them almost perpendicular to the floor. Bend the elbows and pull the arms down until the elbows are at the same height as the shoulders. Make sure to keep the core tight for stability.

Modifications:

- Slower Back Extension Pull Downs
- Faster Back Extension Pull Downs
- Pulsing Back Extension Pull Downs

Muscles Being Worked:

- Back
- Core
- Shoulders
- Arms

Upper Body Exercises

Plank Rows

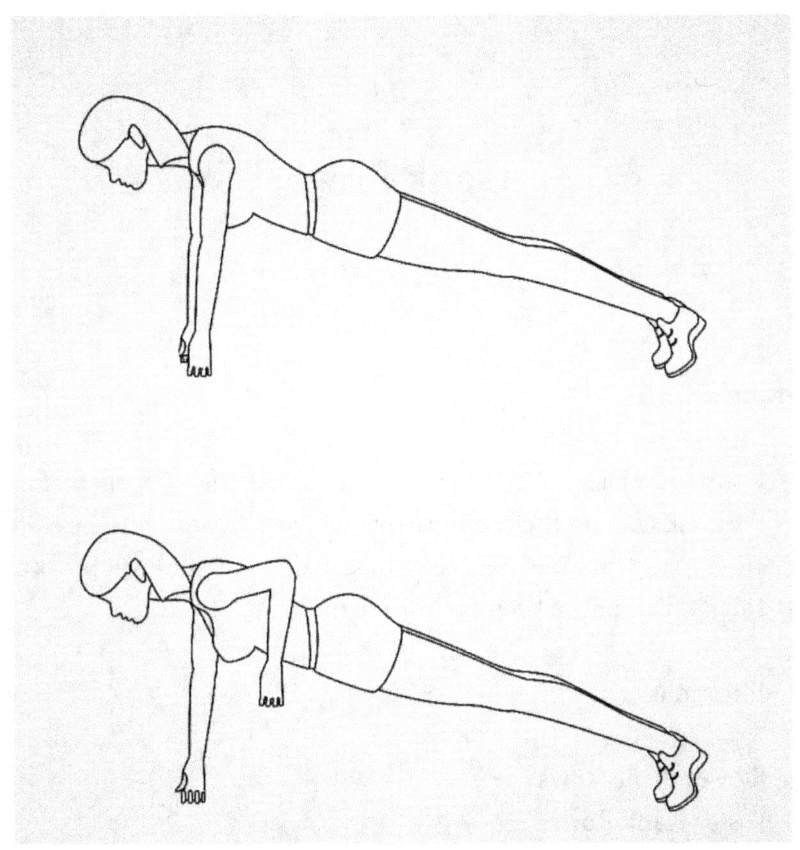

Plank Rows

How to:

- Get into a plank position on the ground with the toes together and the hands flat on the ground. Row one arm up keeping the elbow close to the torso. Bring the arm back down. Repeat on the other side. Make sure to keep the core tight for stability.

Modifications:

- Slower Plank Rows
- Faster Plank Rows
- Place the toes hip width apart instead of together
- Drop down to the knees instead of the toes
- For a challenge, do this movement, but only have one toe on the ground and the other leg up

Muscles Being Worked:

- Core
- Chest
- Arms

Upper Body Exercises

Body Tricep Dips

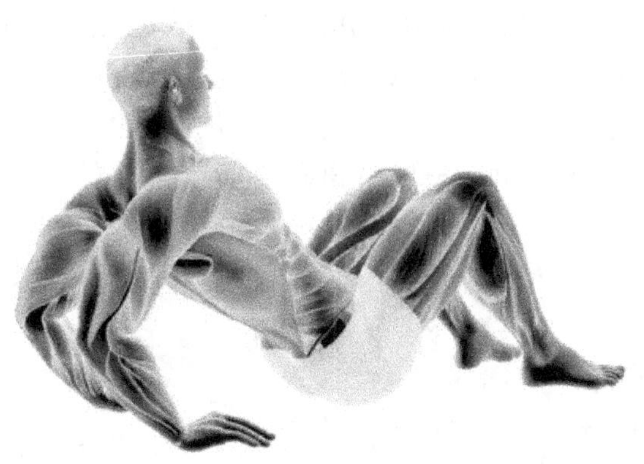

Body Tricep Dips

How to:

- Sit on the ground with the knees bent and behind you, underneath the shoulders, have the arms bent and hands flat on the ground pointing towards the same area as the toes. Raise the butt off the ground to only have the feet and hands touching the floor. Extend the arms until they are straight while keeping the butt off the ground. Lower yourself back down to the starting position. Keep the back as straight as possible throughout the exercise. Make sure to also keep the core tight for stability.

Modifications:

- Slower Body Tricep Dips
- Faster Body Tricep Dips

Muscles Being Worked:

- Arms
- Back

Upper Body Exercises

Walkout

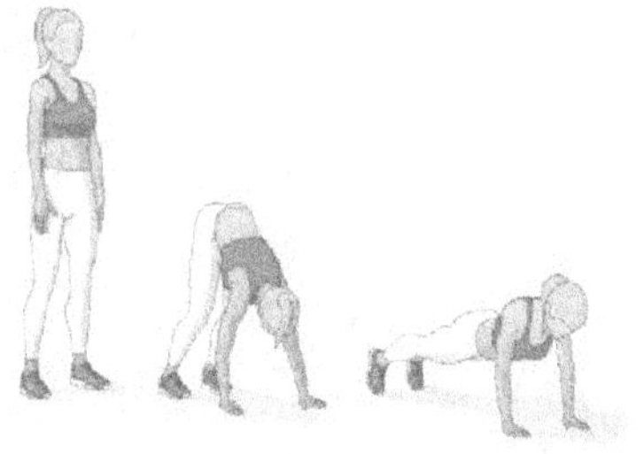

Walkout

How to:

- Start in a standing position with the feet hip width apart. Hinge at the hips and walk the hands from near the feet out away from the body until the body is in a plank position. Reverse the movement by walking the hands back towards the body and unhinging the hips to come back to a standing position

Modifications:

- Slower Walkout
- Faster Walkout
- Add a push up once at the plank position
- Add shoulder taps when at the plank position

Muscles Being Worked:

- Arms
- Chest
- Back
- Core

Upper Body Exercises

Side Plank Rotations

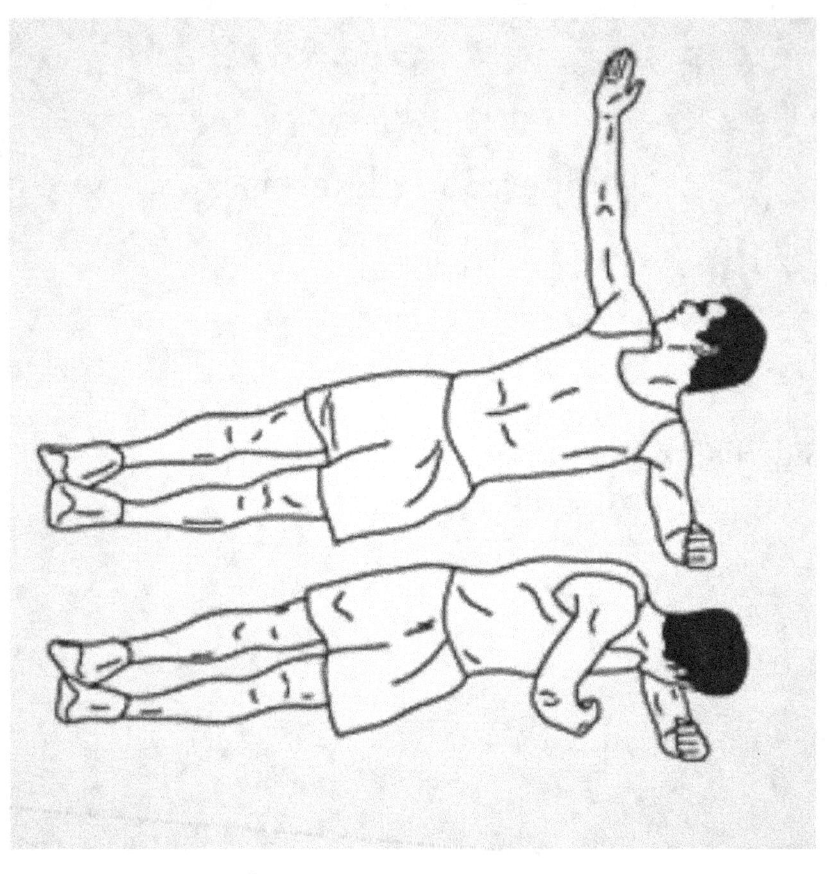

Side Plank Rotations

How to:

- Start in a side plank position with the right shoulder over the elbow. Make sure to keep the entire body in a straight line and reach the left hand to the ceiling. Twist the core forward until the left hand is placed underneath the body. Come back up to the starting position. Make sure to switch sides. Keep the core tight for stability

Modifications:

- Slower Side Plank Rotations
- Faster Side Plank Rotations
- Side plank with the arm extending towards the ceiling and hold

Muscles Being Worked:

- Core
- Back
- Shoulders

Upper Body Exercises

Prone Reverse Fly

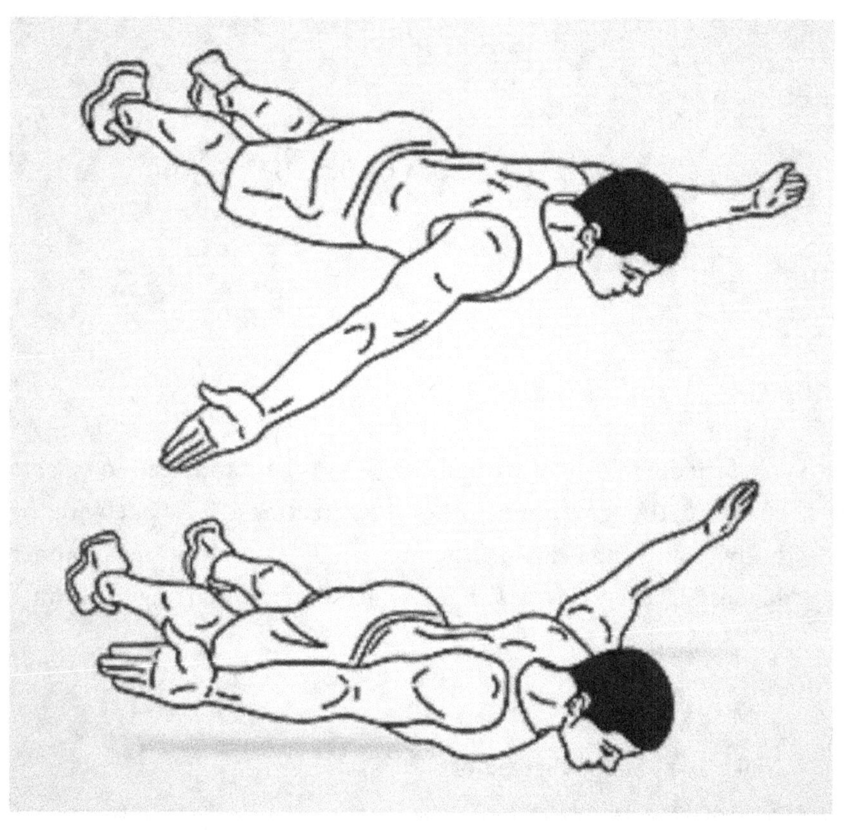

Prone Reverse Fly

How to:

- Lie face down on the ground. Raise the chest and head to be able to extend the arms out to either side, creating a "T" shape with the body. Raise the arms off the ground by squeezing the shoulder blades together. Lower the arms back down to starting position

Modifications:

- Make a "Y" Shape Instead of a "T"
- Slower Prone Reverse Fly
- Faster Prone Reverse Fly

Muscles Being Worked:

- Back

Upper Body Exercises

Standing Lawnmower Pulls

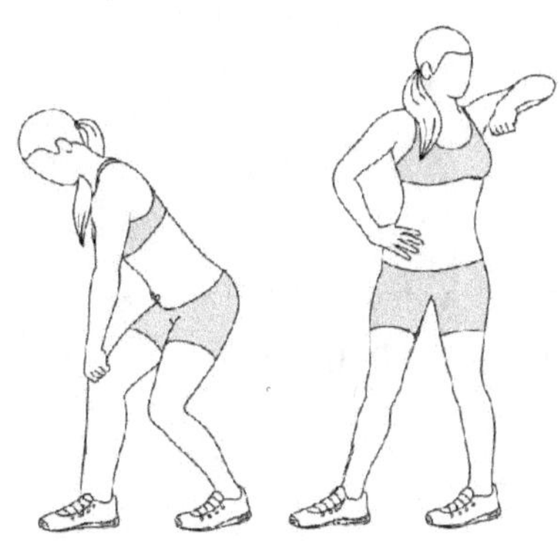

Standing Lawnmower Pulls

How to:

- Stand up straight with the feet shoulder width apart. Squat down and rotate the core so the right hand will almost touch the floor to the left of the left foot. Stand up and rotate the core back to the normal standing position with the hand in front of the right shoulder

Modifications:

- Slower Standing Lawn Mower Pulls
- Faster Standing Lawn Mower Pulls

Muscles Being Worked:

- Core
- Arms
- Shoulders
- Back
- Legs

Lower Body Exercises

Lunges

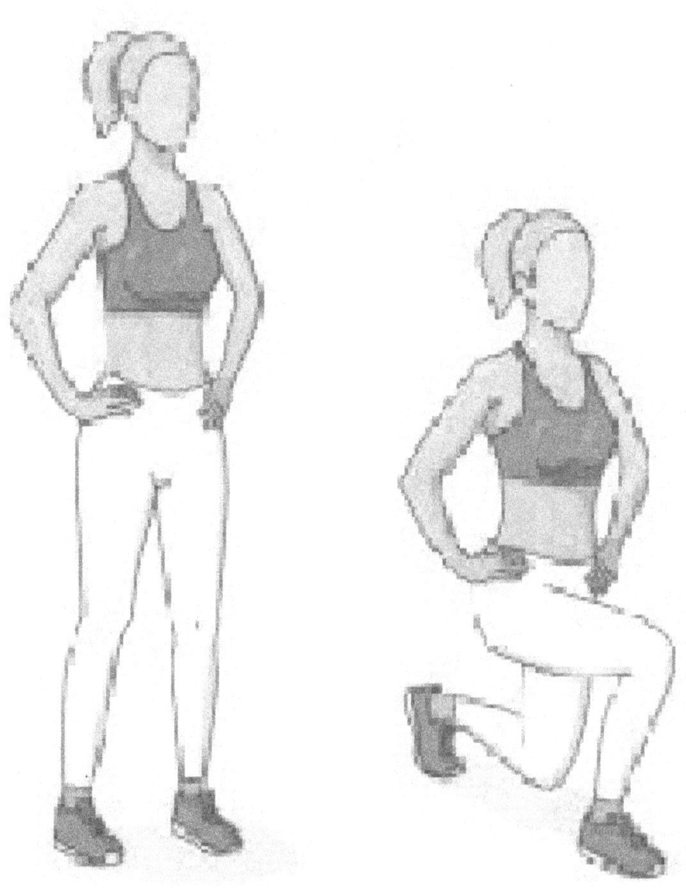

Lunges

How to:

- Stand with the right foot about 2 or 3 feet in front of the left foot. Keep the core tight and posture straight. Bend the knees and lower the body until the left knee is a few inches from the floor. The right thigh should be parallel to the floor at this point, with the weight evenly distributed between both legs. Push back up to the starting position. Make sure to switch sides

Modifications:

- Slower Lunges
- Faster Lunges
- Forward or Backward Lunges
- Walking Lunges
- Pulsing Lunges

Muscles Being Worked:

- Legs
- Core

Lower Body Exercises

Squats

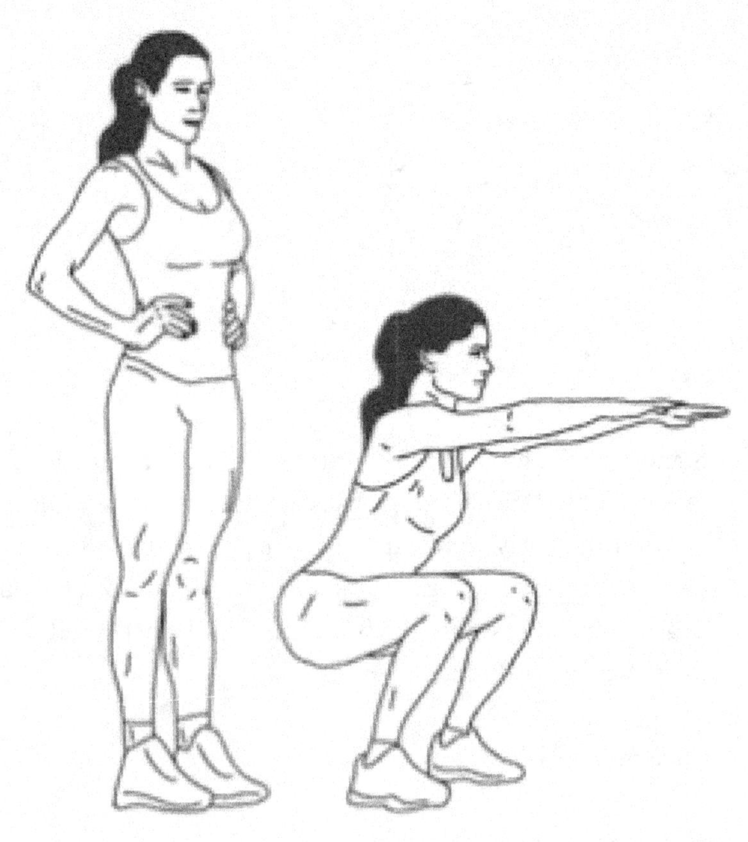

Squats

How to:

- Stand with the feet a little wider than hip width apart with the toes facing front. Drive the hips back while bending the knee. Keep the toes and heels on the ground with the chest up and shoulders back. At the bottom of the squat, the knees should be at about a 90 degree angle. Press into the floor through the heels and return to the standing position.

Modifications:

- Slower Squats
- Faster Squats
- Pulsing Squats
- Single Leg Squats
- Walking Squats

Muscles Being Worked:

- Legs
- Core

Lower Body Exercises

Bridges

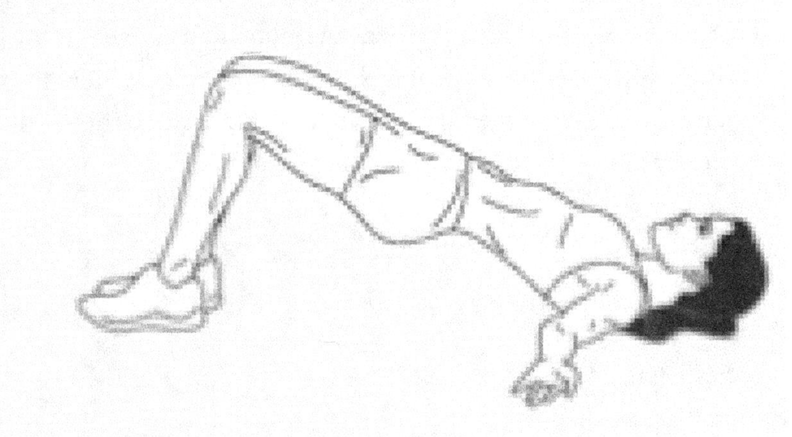

Bridges

How to:

- Lay down with the back touching the floor, knees bent and the feet flat on the ground. The feet should be about hip width apart with the toes pointing straight. The heels of the feet should be about 6-8 inches away from the glutes. Arms are out by the sides with the palms facing the ceiling. Squeeze the glutes and core to lift the hips towards the ceiling. Do not arch the back, the body should be in a straight line from the knee through the hips and to the shoulders. Slowly lower the hips down to the floor.

Modifications:

- Slower Bridges
- Faster Bridges
- Pulsing Bridges
- Single Leg Bridges

Muscles Being Worked:

- Legs

Lower Body Exercises

Calf Raises

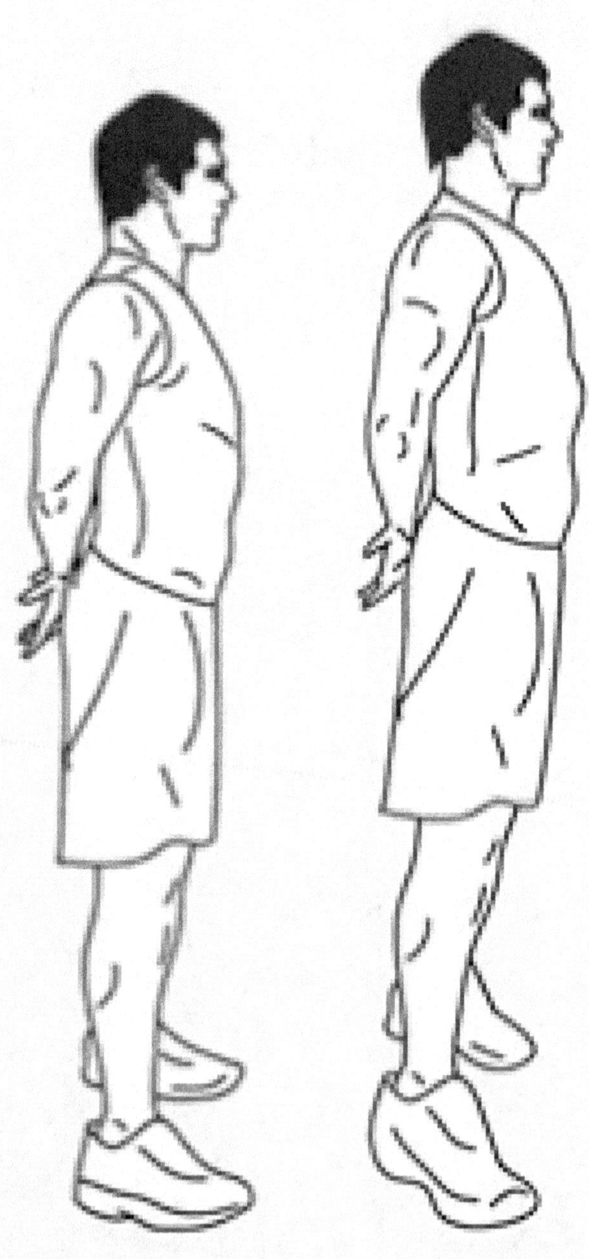

47

Calf Raises

How to:

- Start in a standing position with the feet shoulder width apart and toes pointing forward. Raise the heels off the ground slowly with the knees extended but not locked. Lower the heels back down to the ground, returning to the standing position.

Modifications:

- Slower Calf Raises
- Faster Calf Raises
- Pulsing Calf Raises
- Holding Calf Raises
- Single Leg Calf Raises

Muscles Being Worked:

- Calves

Lower Body Exercises

Plank Jacks

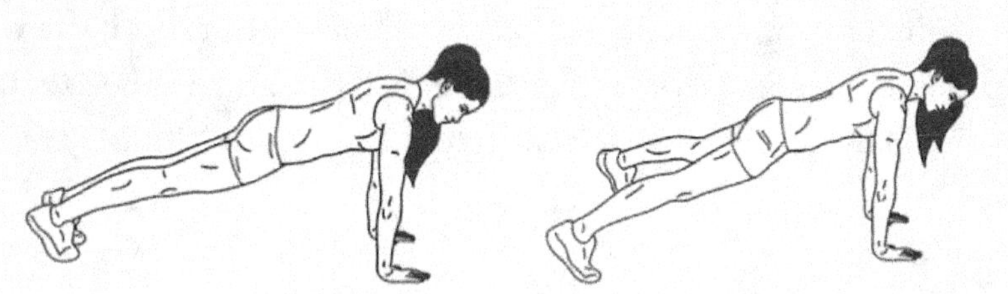

Plank Jacks

How to:

- Start in the plank position on the ground. The arms are extended and hands under the shoulders with the feet together. Make sure to keep the body in a straight line. Keep the core, back and glutes tight for stability. Jump both feet out at the same time as if you were doing a jumping jack with the lower half of your body horizontally. Jump the feet back in, returning to the starting position.

Modifications:

- Slower Plank Jacks
- Faster Plank Jacks
- Walking Out the Jack Instead of Jumping it Out

Muscles Being Worked:

- Legs
- Core
- Back

Lower Body Exercises

Side Leg Raises

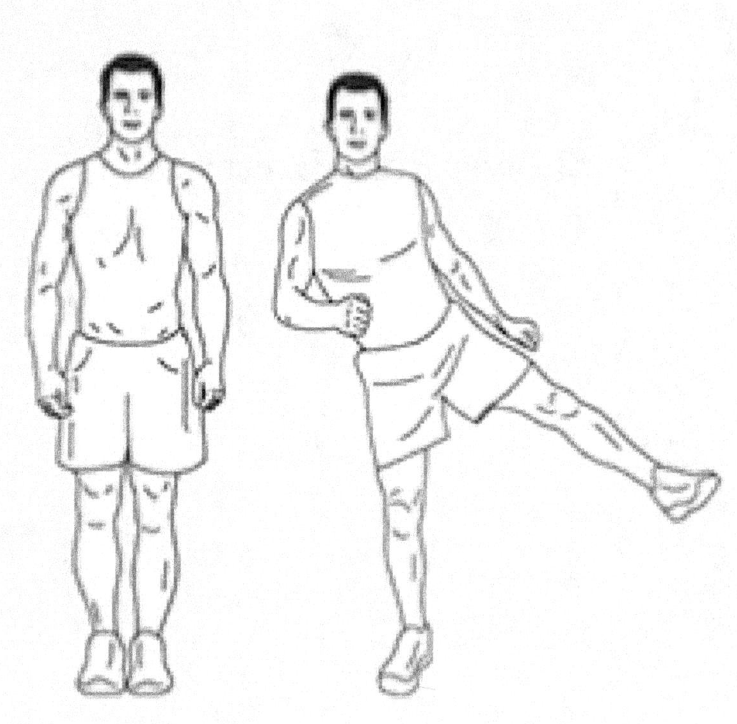

Side Leg Raises

How to:

- Start in a standing position with the feet together with the hands either on the hips or at the sides. Lift the right leg up off the ground laterally, as if you have 2 walls almost touching you; one in front of you and one behind you. Flex the right foot as it is going up and shift the weight onto the left leg. Return to the starting position. Make sure to repeat with the left leg.

Modifications:

- Slower Side Leg Raises
- Faster Side Leg Raises
- Side Leg Raise and Hold
- Side Leg Raise and Pulse

Muscles Being Worked:

- Legs
- Core

Lower Body Exercises

Kneeling to Squat

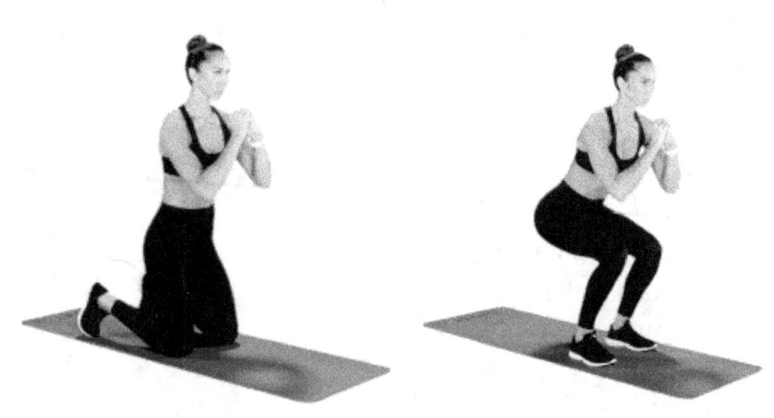

Kneeling to Squat

How to:

- Begin in the kneeling position with the knees hip width apart and the hands together at the front of the chest with the shoulders down. Transfer the weight to the left knee and bring the right foot up and forward into the squat position. Push through the right heel to shift the weight and bring the left foot up and forward into the squatting position. The feet should now be flat on the ground and the thighs parallel to the floor. Transfer the weight to the left foot and step the right foot back into the kneeling position. Shift the weight to the right knee and bring the left leg back into the kneeling position.

Modifications:

- Slower Kneeling to Squats
- Faster Kneeling to Squats
- Kneeling to Squat Jumps (Use arms for momentum)

Muscles Being Worked:

- Legs
- Core

Lower Body Exercises

Side Lunges

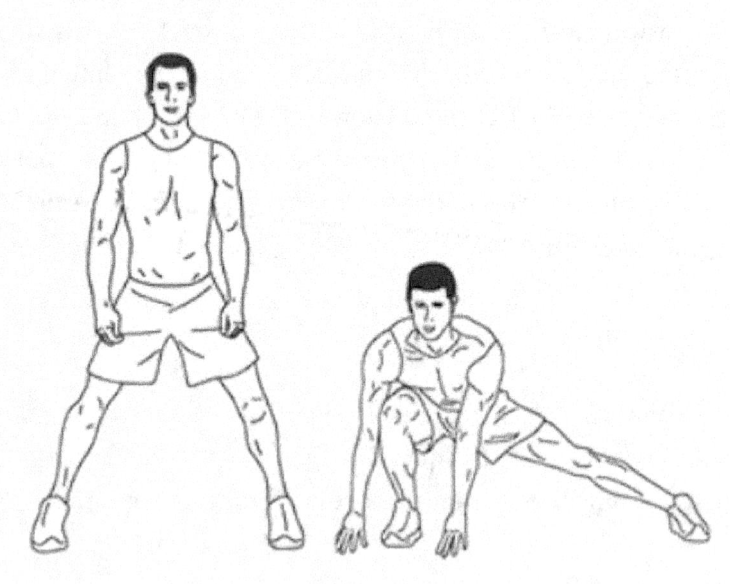

Side Lunges

How to:

- Start in a standing position with the feet wider than the hips. Bend the left knee and drive the hips backward. Pretend as if you are trying to sit on a chair with only the left side of the body. Try to touch the hands to the ground at the bottom. Keep the core tight for stability. In this position the left thigh should be about parallel to the ground. Push through the left heel to drive yourself back up to the starting position. Repeat with the right side.

Modifications:

- Slow Side Lunges
- Fast Side Lunges
- Pulsing Side Lunges
- Repeating Leg Side Lunge (Do Side Leg Lunges on One Leg for Multiple Reps, Then Do the Other Leg)

Muscles Being Worked:

- Legs
- Core

Lower Body Exercises

Fire Hydrants

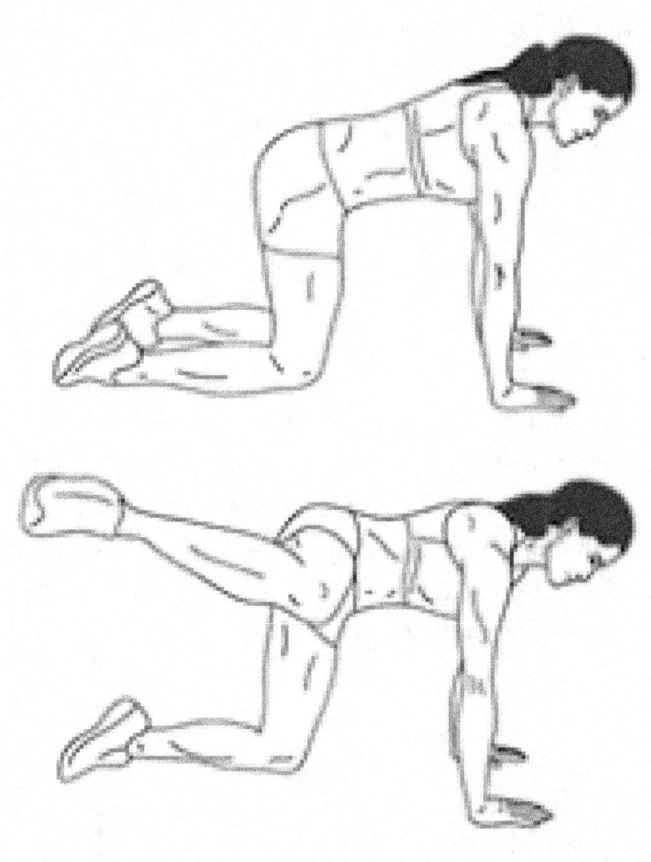

Fire Hydrants

How to:

- Start in a comfortable position with the hands and knees on the ground. Lift one knee off the ground by moving it out to the side and toward the ceiling. Keep the knee bent at a 90 degree angle during the movement. Slowly bring the knee back down to the ground to the starting position. Repeat with the other knee. Keep the core tight for stability.

Modifications:

- Slower Fire Hydrants
- Faster Fire Hydrants
- Pulsing Fire Hydrants
- Add An Extension Of the Leg At The Top of The Fire Hydrant

Muscles Being Worked:

- Legs
- Core
- Back

Lower Body Exercises

Side Kicks

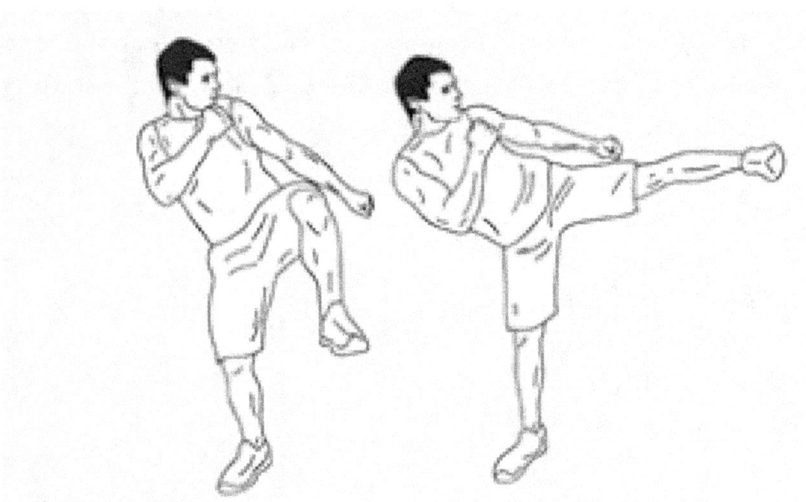

Side Kicks

How to:

- Start in a standing position with the feet about hip width apart. Lift the left knee with the knee bent in front of the body. Drive the knee and foot out, extending the knee and "striking" the target. Keep the core tight for stability. Bring the knee back inwards and back to a bent position. Lastly, bring the foot back down to the starting position. Repeat using the other leg.

Modifications:

- Slower Side Kicks
- Faster Side Kicks
- Jump Side Kicks
- Low Side Kicks

Muscles Being Worked:

- Legs
- Core

Core Exercises

Leg Raises

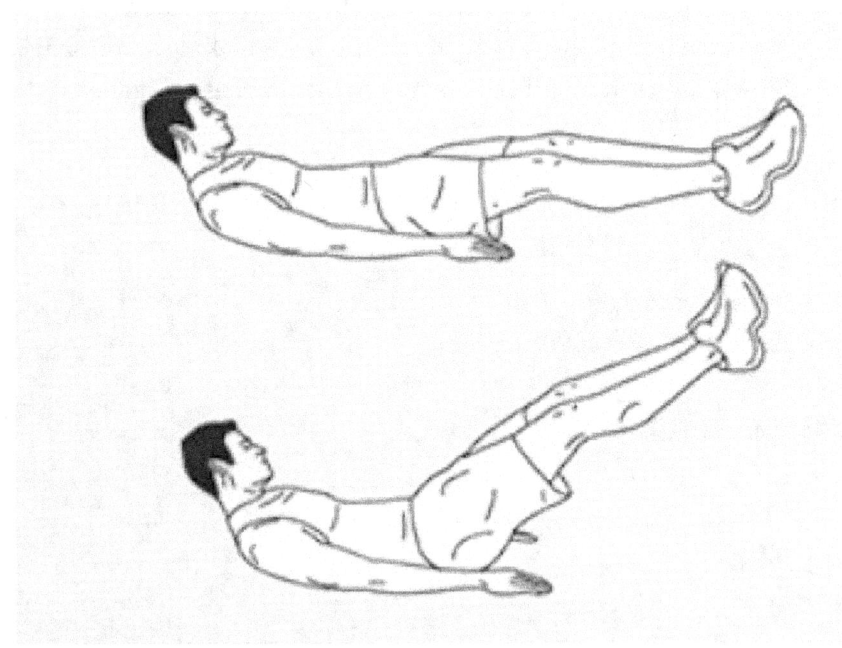

Leg Raises

How to:

- Lie flat on the ground and do a crunch but only with the upper body. Hold at the top. Next, with the legs extended and thighs touching, lift both legs from the floor and keep the legs as straight as possible. Bring the legs all the way up until the body is making an "L" shape. Slowly lower the legs back down into the starting position.

Modifications:

- Slower Leg Raises
- Faster Leg Raises
- Bend the Knees at 90 Degrees

Muscles Being Worked:

- Core
- Back
- Legs

Core Exercises

Flutter Kicks

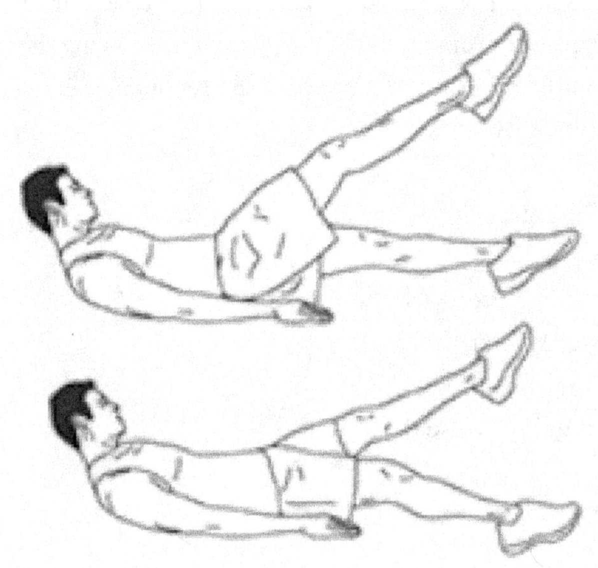

Flutter Kicks

How to:

- Lie on the floor on the back. Do a crunch with the upper body and bring the legs up to about a 45 degree angle. Keep the legs as straight as possible and together. Start to lower one leg towards the ground. Almost touch the ground, then bring the leg back up to meet the other leg. Repeat with the second leg. Keep the core tight for stability.

Modifications:

- Slower Flutter Kicks
- Faster Flutter Kicks

Muscles Being Worked:

- Core

Core Exercises

30 Second Elbow Plank

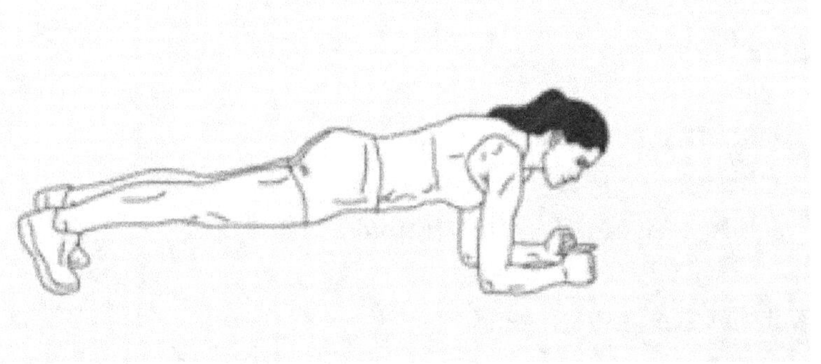

30 Second Elbow Plank

How to:

- Get in a push up position, but bend the arms at the elbows so the weight is on the forearms, not the hands. Tighten the core for stability and hold for 30 seconds.

Modifications:

- Shorter Time Elbow Plank
- Longer Time Elbow Plank
- Lift an Arm Off Of the Ground

Muscles Being Worked:

- Core
- Back
- Arms
- Legs

Core Exercises

Heel Touches

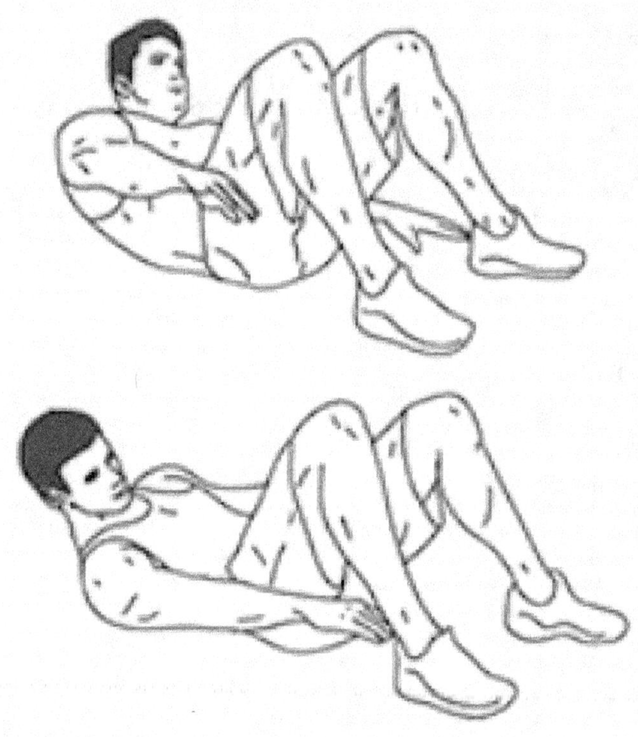

Heel Touches

How to:

- Start on the floor and lie down on the back. Make sure the feet are separated and flat on the floor with the knees bent. Arms should be extended at the sides with the fingers pointing downward. Lift the head to crunch upwards and hold this position. Reach one hand at a time towards the heels in a side bend motion. Continue to alternate

Modifications:

- Slower Heel Touches
- Faster Heel Touches

Muscles Being Worked:

- Core

Core Exercises

Scissor Kicks

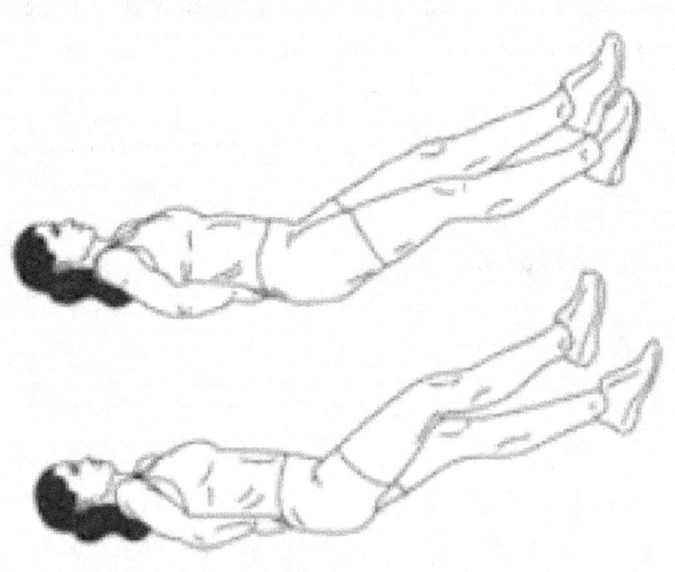

Scissor Kicks

How to:

- Lie on the back with the arms down at the sides or under the small of the back. Lift both legs until they make a 45 degree angle. Keeping both legs straight, make a "V" shape with the legs still at the 45 degree angle. Then bring the legs together, crossing them over each other. Crossing the left leg over the right leg. Widen the legs again to the "V" shape. Bring the legs together to cross each other again, but this time with the right leg over the left leg. Continue alternating. Keep the core tight during the entire exercise.

Modifications:

- Slower Scissor Kicks
- Faster Scissor Kicks

Muscles Being Worked:

- Core

Core Exercises

Crunches

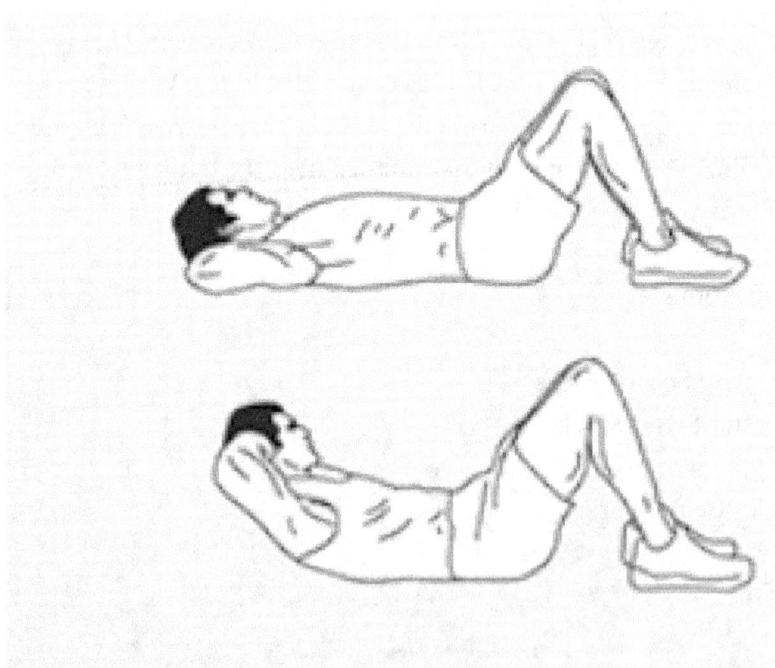

Crunches

How to:

- Lie down on the back with the feet on the floor, hip width apart, and the knees bent. Place your havens behind your neck to help comfort the neck. Contract the core and lift the upper body, keeping the head and neck relaxed. Return slowly back down to the starting position.

Modifications:

- Slower Crunches
- Faster Crunches

Muscles Being Worked:

- Core

Core Exercises

Windshield Wipers

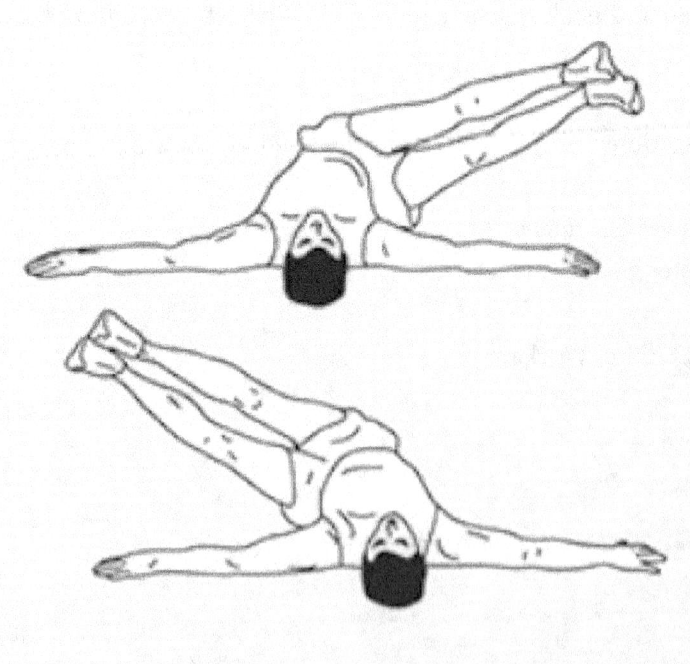

Windshield Wipers

How to:

- Lie on the back with the arms straight out to the sides. Lift the legs so the body is in an "L" Shape. Rotate the hips to one side, keeping the legs as straight as possible, without letting the legs touch the floor. Rotate the hips again to bring the legs back to the starting position. Rotate the hips to the other side, again, without letting the legs touch the ground. Then, return to the starting position.

Modifications:

- Slower Windshield Wipers
- Faster Windshield Wipers
- Bend the Knees at 90 Degree Angle for an Easier Modification

Muscles Being Worked:

- Core

Core Exercises

High Knees

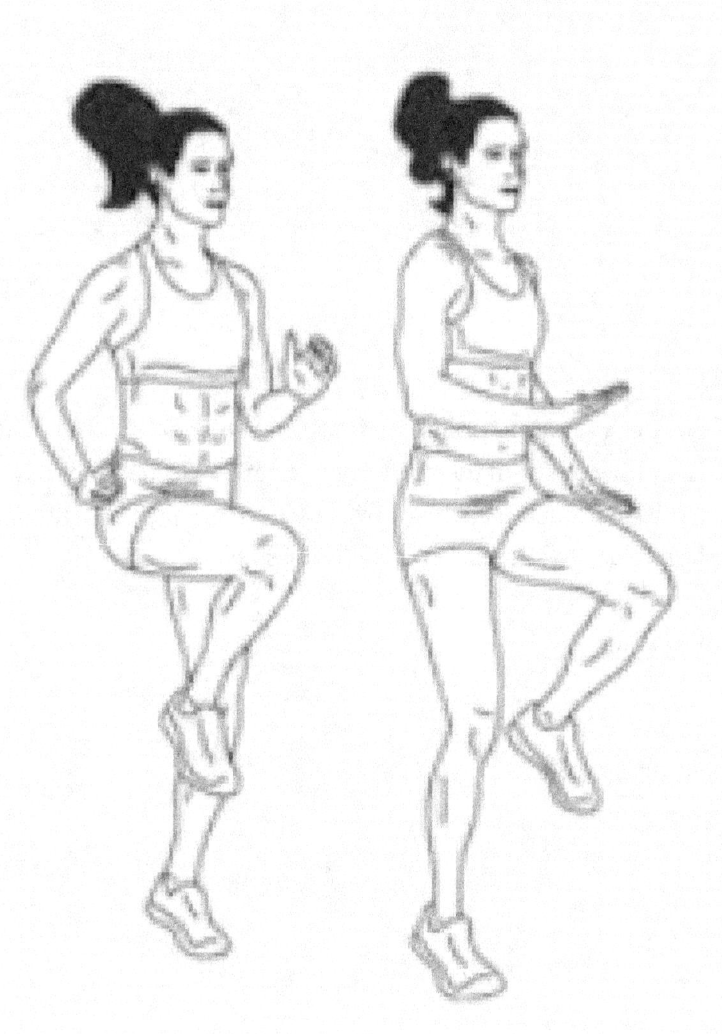

High Knees

How to:

- Start in a standing position with the feet hip width apart. Bring the right knee up until the right thigh is parallel to the floor. Bring the left leg back down to the starting position. Repeat using the left leg. Make sure to keep the core tight for stability

Modifications:

- Slower High Knees
- Faster High Knees

Muscles Being Worked:

- Core
- Legs

Core Exercises

Side Plank Dips

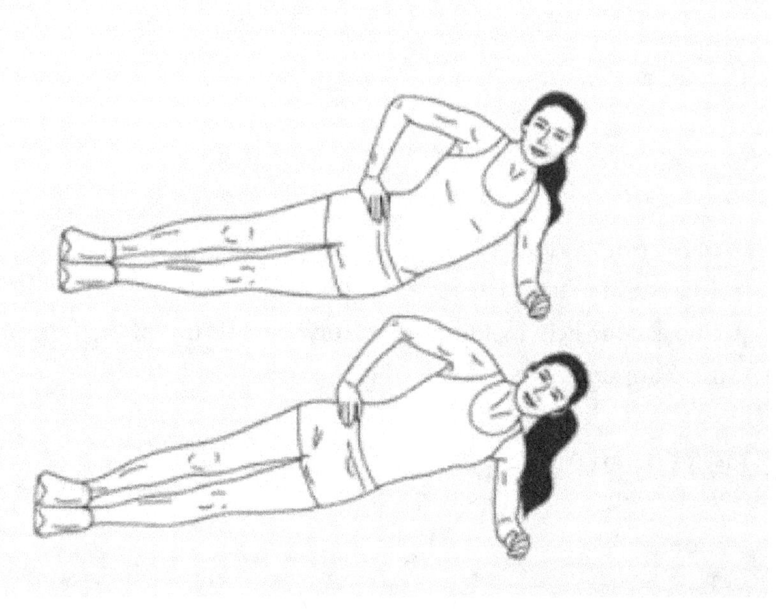

Side Plank Dips

How to:

- Lie on the side with the feet stacked on top of each other. Position the elbow under the shoulder. Lift the body off the ground by driving the hips towards the ceiling. Make sure to switch sides to get an even workout. Keep the core tight and move slowly and with control.

Modifications:

- Slower Side Plank Dips
- Faster Side Plank Dips
- Stagger the Feet by Placing the Top Leg in Front of the Bottom Leg for Support

Muscles Being Worked:

- Core
- Back
- Shoulders
- Legs

Core Exercises

Ab Bicycles

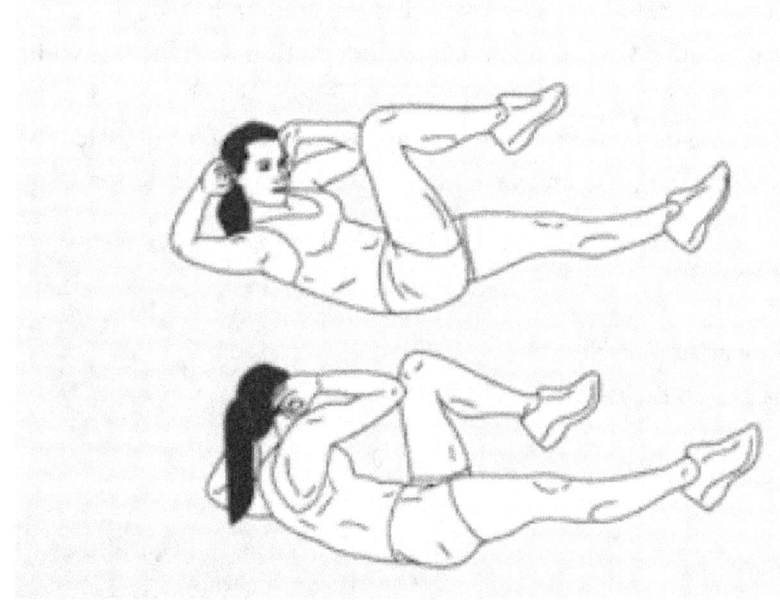

Ab Bicycles

How to:

- Lie flat on the floor with the lower back pressed to the ground and the knees bent with the feet on the floor and the hands behind the head. Squeeze the core muscle to hold the head and shoulders off the ground. Raise the knees until there is about a 90 degree angle being made. Go through the bicycling motion with the legs while at the same time rotating the core. The opposite knee should be touching or almost touching the opposite elbow. Alternate sides by twisting the torso and switching legs.

Modifications:

- Slower Ab Bicycles
- Faster Ab Bicycles

Muscles Being Worked:

- Core
- Legs
- Back

Conclusion

In the journey of fitness, the exploration of bodyweight exercises for both the upper and lower body has unveiled a realm of possibilities that extend far beyond the confines of traditional workout routines. We are empowered by the knowledge that our own bodies are the most versatile and accessible tools for fitness.

In the pursuit of a fit body, we've discovered that bodyweight exercises offer many benefits. By harnessing the resistance of our own weight, we have the opportunity to cultivate functional strength that translates seamlessly into everyday activities. From the graceful pull of a push-up to the explosive energy of a plank jack, each exercise has the potential to sculpt muscles, enhance endurance, and contribute to a well-rounded physique. Additionally, this book has emphasized the versatility and adaptability of bodyweight exercises. Regardless of fitness level or location, the potential to engage in these movements remains constant. The absence of expensive equipment or gym memberships ensures that anyone, anywhere can embark on a journey towards fitness.

In conclusion, this book stands as a testament to the transformative potential of bodyweight exercises for the upper and lower body. The path to a healthier, more fulfilled life awaits—one bodyweight movement at a time.

Remember, many bodyweight exercises engage multiple muscle groups simultaneously, so don't be afraid to mix and match exercises from different categories to create comprehensive full-body workouts. Always focus on proper form and gradually progress to more challenging variations as you become more proficient in each exercise.

If you found this book helpful, please leave a review on Amazon

Resources

The advantages of body-weight exercise. Harvard Health. (2022, February 15). https://www.health.harvard.edu/exercise-and-fitness/the-advantages-of-body-weight-exercise

The art of shadowboxing: Why we shadowbox. Gloveworx. (n.d.). https://www.gloveworx.com/blog/shadowboxing-part-one/#:~:text=while%20in%20movement.-,Exercise,build%2Dup%20some%20muscle%20mass.

Bedosky, L. (2023, March 27). *How to do Scissor Kicks*. BODi. https://www.beachbodyondemand.com/blog/scissor-kicks

Bodyweight prone reverse fly. Thrive Personal Training. (n.d.). https://thrivept.net/exercises/body-weight-prone-reverse-fly/

Bone, M. and J. T. (2023, April 24). *6 leg lift exercises to strengthen your core*. Cleveland Clinic. https://health.clevelandclinic.org/how-to-do-leg-lifts/

Burn, D. (2022, February 17). *How to side plank dip like a pro*. Life by Daily Burn. https://dailyburn.com/life/fitness/how-to-side-plank-dip-like-a-pro/

Chelsea Evers, N.-C. (2022, May 1). *How to do standing calf raises: Techniques, benefits, variations.* Verywell Fit. https://www.verywellf it.com/how-to-do-calf-raises-4801090

Chertoff, J. (2019, May 23). *Plank jacks: How-to, benefits, safety tips, and more.* Healthline. https://www.healthline.com/health/exercise-fitness/ plank-jacks#how-to

Daisy. (2021a, June 1). *Arm circles: Illustrated exercise guide.* SPOTEBI. https://www.spotebi.com/exercise-guide/arm-circles/

Daisy. (2021b, June 3). *Windshield wipers: Illustrated exercise guide.* SPOTEBI. https://www.spotebi.com/exercise-guide/windshield-w ipers/

Daisy. (2021c, June 5). *Inchworm: Illustrated exercise guide.* SPOTEBI. https://www.spotebi.com/exercise-guide/inchworm/#:~:text=The%2 0inchworm%20is%20a%20great,increases%20your%20balance%20and %20stability.

Daisy. (2021d, June 19). *Lawnmower pull: Illustrated exercise guide.* SPOTEBI. https://www.spotebi.com/exercise-guide/lawnmower-pull /#:~:text=The%20lawnmower%20pull%20is%20a,helps%20to%20defin e%20your%20waist.

Daisy. (2021e, June 24). *Side Plank Rotation: Illustrated Exercise Guide.* SPOTEBI. https://www.spotebi.com/exercise-guide/side-plank-rotati on/

Elizabeth Quinn, M. (2023, May 26). *How to do a bicycle crunch: Techniques, benefits, variations.* Verywell Fit. https://www.verywellf

it.com/bicycle-crunch-exercise-3120058

Everything you need to know about reps and sets. Everything You Need to Know About Reps and Sets | Planet Fitness. (n.d.). https://www.planetfitness.com/community/articles/everything-you-need-know-about-reps-and-sets#:~:text=A%20%22rep%2C%22%20short%20for,help%20you%20effectively%20pace%20yourself.

Fire hydrant exercise: Tips and recommended variations. hingehealth. (n.d.). https://www.hingehealth.com/resources/articles/fire-hydrants/

Floor tricep dips – how to video, Alternatives & More. – How To Video, Alternatives & More. (n.d.). https://www.fitnessai.com/exercise/floor-tricep-dips

How to do a plank row. ClassPass. (n.d.-a). https://classpass.com/movements/plank-row

How to do Flutter Kicks. ClassPass. (n.d.-b). https://classpass.com/movements/flutter-kicks

How to do high knees. ClassPass. (n.d.-c). https://classpass.com/movements/high-knees

Jones, J. P. (2023, July 20). *5 ways to do a side kick.* wikiHow. https://www.wikihow.com/Do-A-Side-Kick

Kneel to squat. SWEAT. (n.d.). https://www.sweat.com/blogs/exercises/kneel-to-squat

Luna, D. (2023, April 17). *The lat pulldown: Benefits, muscles worked, etc..*

Inspire US. https://www.inspireusafoundation.org/lat-pulldown/

Mahaffey, K. (n.d.). *How to do a glute bridge: Form, workouts, and more.* NASM. https://blog.nasm.org/how-to-do-a-glute-bridge

Mayo Foundation for Medical Education and Research. (2021, October 6). *The right way to warm up and cool down.* Mayo Clinic. https://www.mayoclinic.org/healthy-lifestyle/fitness/in-depth/exercise/art-200455 17

Muinos, L. (2021, October 17). *How to do side lunges: Techniques, benefits, variations.* Verywell Fit. https://www.verywellfit.com/how-to-do-side-lunges-techniques-benefits-variations-5186818

Neumann, K. D., & Seaver, M. (2023, March 8). *How to do squats (video): Proper squat form anyone can master.* Real Simple. https://www.realsimple.com/health/fitness-exercise/workouts/squat-form

The New York Times. (n.d.). *How to do a forearm plank.* The New York Times. https://www.nytimes.com/guides/well/activity/how-to-do-a-forearm-plank

Nunez, K. (2019, September 26). *How to do crunches safely and other exercise options for toned ABS.* Healthline. https://www.healthline.com/health/exercise-fitness/how-to-do-crunches

Paige Waehner, C. (2022, November 25). *How to lunge: Techniques, benefits, variations.* Verywell Fit. https://www.verywellfit.com/how-to-lunge-variations-modifications-and-mistakes-1231320

Pushups. Physiopedia. (n.d.). https://www.physio-pedia.com/Pushups#

:~:text=From%20a%20prone%20position%2C%20the,body%20until%2
0arm%20is%20extended.

Safe exercise - orthoinfo - aaos. OrthoInfo. (n.d.). https://orthoinfo.aaos.
org/en/staying-healthy/safe-exercise/

Set, S. F. (2021, December 9). *Heel touches: Correct form, muscles worked,
& alternatives*. SET FOR SET. https://www.setforset.com/blogs/news/
heel-touches